Pranayama Healing: How To Use Pranayama For Self Healing And Have Healthy Body And Mind

CHAPTER

Introduction

Benefits of Pranayama

Pranayama as a Tool to Counter Stress

Pranayama for Depression And Anxiety

Techniques of Pranayama

Conclusion

DISCLAIMER: This book is not intended to be a substitute for the medical advice of a licensed

physician. The reader should consult with their doctor in any matters relating to his/her health.

Before beginning any new exercise program it is recommended that you seek medical advice

from your personal physician.

Introduction

Breath is indispensable to life. It is the very first thing we start with when we enter this world that is taking birth and stop it when we leave this world that is death. In between birth and death, we breathe about a billion times. What we may not understand is that the mind, body, and breath are closely associated and can impact each other. Our breathing is impacted by our considerations, and our contemplations and physiology can be affected by our breath. Figuring out how to inhale deliberately and with consciousness can be an important instrument in re-establishing harmony in the mind and body.

Prana, active by nature, gets to be distinctly sluggish in our rigid bodies with cramped lungs as well as body muscles that we pick not to move in our love for apparatuses, inactive ways of life, and addictive comfy foods that inflate our bodies and deaden our minds.

Away from the standards of natural breathing, there is, in addition, a knack to taming your breath in more commanding ways. The lessons of yoga, martial arts and numerous other enlightening and pious systems have bottomless roots in breath nurturing. in accordance with the majority of these ancient lessons, breathing creates electromagnetic energy or life force energy —generally known as Prana, Qi or Mana— which can recuperate your body and extend your religious practices.

Pranayama is a portion of Yoga that educates you the skill of stretching your breath in a wide range of ways. While rehearsing pranayama the breath ought to be skillfully breathed in, breathed out and held back. It shows you to change the intensity, velocity, and form of breathing.

Pranayama is a Sanskrit word which truly converts into 'expansion of the prana or breath'. "Prana" implies life-force and it is the essence or indispensable energy that infuses the body. Prana is the connection amongst brain and perception. The physical expression of 'prana' is breath and 'ayama' intends to a degree or prolong the breath.

Actually pranayama are the breathing exercises which were developed by the ancient yogis. Pranayama has been practiced for thousand years in India by yogis. Pranayama is a scientific breathing process where control over prana (breath) is achieved.

Benefits of Pranayama:

Advantages of pranayama are both substantial and elusive. God has given prana, the preeminent wellspring of power freely to every individual. Appropriate use of this free wellspring of energy can roll out surprising improvements to our health, energy, and self-assurance. We can't merely associate prana with oxygen that is present in the air; the air we inhale is likewise full of crucial energy that is prana. All advantages of pranayama can't be composed; there are loads of delicate alterations like the peace of mind as well as clear thoughts that transpire in our mind. Pranayama is being practiced regularly in whole world and a lot of benefits are being discovered from practicing pranayama. When you start practicing pranayama you will not even know how many of your illnesses are being cured which you don't even know about in your body. Pranayama has been found to cure even cancer like diseases, so there is no excuse to not to practice pranayama. If you have any illness, I recommend you to practice pranayama for your illness. Even if you don't have any illness, even then I recommend you to practice pranayama because after started doing pranayama you will never fall sick. This is the power of practicing pranayama. Millions of people starts their day with pranayama. Give your day's 30 minutes to pranayama and I assure you that the rest of your day will be so beautiful, peaceful, your mind will be so relaxed and your body will feel so energized. 30 minutes of 24 hours is a very small fraction of time. If you don't have 30 minutes for your body and mind, I don't think you have life. Benefits of practicing pranayama are countless, practice pranayama and experience it yourself. Here are some important benefits of practicing pranayama:-

Condensed breathing rate

With yoga breathing, you can prepare yourself to inhale more gradually as well as more intensely. You can lessen your breathing rate from around 15 breaths a minute to 5 to 6 breaths a minute, which adds up to decreasing the breathing rate by 33%. Decreased breathing rate pilots to:

- Slowing down the rate of heart as additional oxygen can be pumped-up even with lesser breaths. Follow the ratio of 1:2 for inhalation: exhalation.

- Reduced deterioration of interior organs.

- Lowering of circulatory strain, unwinding of body pressures and calmer nerves.

Longevity of life

Based on the philosophy of yoga, lifespan relies on your breathing rate. You can extend your life span by lowering the rate of your breath. For instance, a tortoise takes 4-5 breaths in a minute and it lives for 200 years or more.

Perks up blood circulation

As a consequence of breathing, the newly oxygenated blood (through inhalation) is transported from the lungs to the heart. The heart pumps it through arteries as well as the veins to the different parts of the body, from where it oozes into each tissue plus cell. This enhances the blood circulation and more oxygen or prana or cosmic energy makes it to each and every part of your body.

Healthy heart

Our heart is the most innovative organ of our body. Our heart beats 100,000 times in a day. It pumps blood throughout the day constantly till you are alive. The health of your heart decides your life longevity and the quality of life in your old age. Thus when there is more oxygen in the blood it entails that more oxygen is supplied to the muscles of the heart.

Benefits of Pranayama to the working of our body organs

- Better working of autonomic framework enhances the working of lungs, diaphragm, heart, intestines, pancreas, abdomen, and kidneys.

- The digestive system enhances and ailments relating to stomach related organs are cured.

- General touchiness because of laziness/weariness vanishes.

- By practicing pranayama the organs of the body receives more oxygen, removal of toxins from the body takes place, and subsequently inception of different ailments is barred. Pranayama reinforces the immune system.

Enhanced mental health

- By practicing pranayama it gives you freedom from any kind of pessimistic as well as injurious psychological states like arrogance, greed for money, depression, prurience, anger etc.

- With pranayama changes of the brain are controlled and it readies the psyche for meditation. By practicing pranayama, you will start feeling the lightness of your body, sense inner peace, enhanced sleep, improved memory, and enhanced concentration whereby bettering the religious powers/ abilities.

Better quality of life in old age

When a person reaches his middle age and if he is inactive in his life then the tissues of the lung become lesser flexible and therefore the capacity of the lungs decreases. Pranayama will surely reduce the impacts of the following problems in old age:

•Loss of energy.

•Accumulation of uric acid in the circulatory system which regularly prompts to successive pains in the joints and uneasiness.

•Backaches, cerebral pains, stiffness, hardening muscles, and joints.

•Proper flow of blood is hindered by a lethargic diaphragm or tempering arteries.

It is prescribed to begin learning pranayama from a yoga instructor immediately so as to experience the massive advantages of pranayama. Advantages of yoga breathing can be acknowledged just by experience. Make it a habit of practicing yoga breathing exercises every day.

Pranayama as a Tool to Counter Stress

When you encounter stressful reflections, your thoughtful sensory system triggers the body's old battle or flight reaction, giving you a burst of energy to react to the apparent risk. Your breathing gets to be distinctly shallow and fast, and you principally inhale from the chest and not the lower lungs. This way you will feel short of breath, which is a typical side effect when you feel nervous or irritated. In the meantime, your body creates a surge of hormones, for example, cortisol and epinephrine (otherwise called adrenaline), which raises your BP and heartbeat rate and places you in a stepped up condition of extreme alert.

If you breathe deeply then you will be able to reverse these side effects in a split second and feel calm both in your mind and body. When you inhale deeply and gradually, you trigger the parasympathetic sensory system, which overturns the stress reaction in your body. When you breathe deeply the vagus nerve is fueled which in turn slows your heart rate, lowers your BP and calms both your mind and body.

Furthermore, when you breathe deeply then you also engage your abdominal muscles as well as the diaphragm rather than the muscles in the upper chest as well as neck area. This habituation of the respiratory muscles effects in the enhanced competence of oxygen replaces with every inhalation by letting more air interchange to take place in the lower lungs which in turn decreases the strain on the muscles of your upper chest as well as neck, and hence these muscles are able to relax. In a nutshell, deep breathing is more soothing and competent, letting higher quantities of oxygen to get to the body's cells plus tissues.

Pranayama helps for healthy and youthful skin

It is one of the most common and visible benefit of pranayama, I don't know how I should convince you for it, but I just want to say that practice it and experience it for yourself. I have myself cured my pimple problems by practicing pranayama and experienced a healthy and glowing skin. Not only me but I have seen many people cured their skin problems by practicing it. And I also think that it could be one of the main reasons, why most people start practicing pranayama, simply because it works.

Pranayama for Depression And Anxiety

There are many ways of treating your depression and anxiety. For example:-

Exercising, Meditation, Medication, Therapies and many more, but you may not realize

that the safest, effective and inexpensive way to treat each of these conditions is in your

hands. It is your own breath .

By controlling their breath (a practice of pranayama), yogis have found that they can

alter their state of mind. The pranayama practices prescribed in this book creates the

effect of slowing down and regularizing your breath. This engages what scientists call

the parasympathetic nervous system, a complex biological mechanism that calms and

soothes us.

For treatment of depression you need not to take any medicine, you just follow practices

prescribed in this book and see the results. You can say it is natural depression

treatment. But why should you listen to me over this advice, because I have seen many

people, seeing tremendous difference in their feelings, who have been told by their doctors that their depression can't be treated. So, it leaves no excuses for you that you

should'nt practice pranayama and see the difference in your life.

Techniques of Pranayama

There are so many of pranayama practices to perform. But nobody have that much time and needs to do that many of practices. Basically, the following pranayama practices covers all the needs and if practiced regularly, then will completely transform your life. You don't have to hassle around to find which practices to perform and which to leave, just perform the practices given below and you will see the difference more than you have expected, Because, many of the benefits of practicing pranayama you will see by yourself, which I have not mentioned in the book, because it is not possible at least for me to describe all the benefits of pranayama.

1. Bhastrika Pranayama

Bhastrika pranayama comprises of deep breathing in and powerfully breathing out. You should practice Bhastrika Pranayama normally for 3-5 minutes twice every day in the fresh air. In this pranayama, the body gets the greatest measure of oxygen because of complete breathing in and breathing out.

Steps

1. Be seated comfortably on the flat ground. If you are not able to sit down then you can sit on a chair as this pranayama is linked to the breath.

2. Take a full breath through both nostrils and fill the lungs with air and afterward, breathe out with a hissing sound.

3. Deeply Inhale completely exhale.

4. Do this for 2 min to 5 minutes max.

2. Kapalbhati Pranayama

Forcefully breathe out so that your stomach goes deep inside. Kapalbhati pranayama cures stomach issue like dyspepsia and constipation and cure heart issues, frees tummy fat and heals acidity

Steps

1. Sit on a flat floor and fold your legs. Keep your spine straight and close your eyes.

2. Keep your right palm on your right knee and the left on the left knee.

3. Now take a full breath and breathe out with all your force so your stomach will go deep inside.

4. When you breathe out with hissing sound then try to believe that your issues are leaving through your nose.

5. Do not stress when you breathe in. there should be no strain when you inhale. Breathing in will be done naturally after each breathing out.

6. Repeat these steps for 5 minutes and rest. You can, later on, increase the time to 15 – 30 minutes.

7. Do not practice very fast. You should practice only at a medium pace.

3. Bahya Pranayama

This pranayama is amazing for curing hernia, prostate issues, acidity and stomach issues. In this pranayama, the breath is kept outside amid the practice so it is called Bahya Pranayama. Bahya signifies "outside". It ought to be done after Kapalbhati pranayama.

Steps

1. Sit in Padmasana or Siddhasana pose.

2. Take a full breath and breathe out totally to clear lungs as far as possible.

3. Hold your breath and touch your chin to the chest and is known as (Jalandhar Bandha or Throat lock). By pulling your stomach in and up under the rib confine with the end goal that the stomach and back appear to touch each other from inside. It is called (Uddiyana Bandha). Lift the muscle from groin region and this is called (Mulabandha or Root bolt).

4. Hold these three locks say for 10-15 seconds breathe in deeply to release these three bandhas.

5. Repeat Bahya pranayama for 2-5 minutes every day.

4. Anulom Vilom Pranayama

Anulom Vilom pranayama is one of the fabulous breathing activities which are otherwise called Nadi Shodhana. The normal practice offers energy to the body and discharges stress and tension. It ought to be practiced in the morning in the open that too in empty stomach. This is a very good breathing activity to enhance blood flow, to remove blocks in the heart. It also helps to release tension, depression, stress and nervousness. It is also effective to control high BP, cures allergy, asthma as well as sinus.

Steps

1. Sit comfortably on the ground but if you can't sit down then sit on a chair.

2. Now close the right nostril with right thumb and inhale through left nostril. After that close left nostril with middle and ring finger and exhale through the right nostril.

3. Now breathe deeply with right nostril and after that close right nostril and exhale deeply with left nostril. Repeat.

4. Do this for 5-10 minutes.

5. Remember that your breathing has to be not in the stomach but up to the lungs.

5. Bhramari Pranayama

The Bhramari pranayama technique of *breathing* has got its name from Bhramari the black Indian bee. Bhramari pranayama is the best breathing activity to calm your mind.

It helps you to release your anger, frustration as well as agitation. Practice every day for 3 to 5 minutes.

Steps

1. Sit straight in Padmasana or Sukhasana and press your tragus with your thumb.

2. Place your forefingers on the temple and with the rest of the fingers close your eyes.

3. Start breathing in through both the nostril deeply and gradually.

4. By closing your mouth make a humming sound like a bee. You can say 'Om' in a very soft and humming sound.

5. Feel your body is releasing all the impurities and you experience positive energy.

6. Udgeeth pranayama

In this pranayama, the breathing in and breathing out span ought to be long. Breathe in deeply and chant 'Ommmmmmmmmm' for quite a while as much you can. It treats hypertension, acidity, and enhances memory power. It is also known as 'Omkara Japa' implying 'Om' chanting. You should practice this technique daily.

Steps

1. Sit in a relaxed and suitable pose.

2. In this pranayama, the breathing in and breathing out duration has to be long.

3. Inhale deeply and when you breathe out keep chanting Ommmmmmmmmm for quite a while.

4. In all pranayama, the breath assumes a critical part. So focus on your breath and feel a positive energy comes when you breathe in and negative energy goes out when you breathe out.

5. Repeat this for 5-10 minutes.

7. Pranav Pranayama and Benefits

This is the last and the seventh pranayama. This technique will help you to concentrate on inhaling and exhaling. It is excellent for meditation as well as increasing your concentration power. It releases stress, depression and fortifies the mind. This is an extremely basic breathing activity. This is also one kind of meditation.

Steps

1. Sit in Padmasana, Sukhasana or Vajrasana silently.

2. Breathe regularly and focus on breathing in and breathing out.

3. While practicing Pranav pranayama envision that God is everywhere and in everything you see.

4. Practice for 3 minutes to 1 hour according to the time available.

Conclusion

Pranayama or breathing activity can be an incredible approach to begin your day. Early morning is the best time to practice pranayama, particularly outside where you can get fresh and natural air. It is better and good for you if you could do the breathing exercises in your empty stomach. While you do Pranayama you have to be absolutely in fineness with your inhalation and exhalation as well as in genuineness of maintenance. Each breath in triggers the Central Nervous System into motivating the tangential nerves and each breath out activates the repeal procedure. While you retain your breath, both procedures happen. While breathing in or holding the breath in pranayama cycle, bear in mind to guarantee that the abdomen is not swelling.

In pranayama breathing, the brain is calm and this permits the sensory system to work all the more successfully. The advantage of pranayama is that brain gets sharp as well as steady and it also increases your concentration power. You can focus your mind on any kind of micro things. The main thing you can learn when you practice Pranayama is to move energy cyclically, vertically as well as horizontally to the borders of your body. Another advantage is that out of triguna-Satvaguna increments and Rajoguna (Wayward), Tamoguna (languid) diminishes. The increment in Satvaguna (seven healthy attributes) is essential for human's spiritual advancement.

****

Printed in Great Britain
by Amazon